THE Complete
AFib Diet Cookbook for Seniors

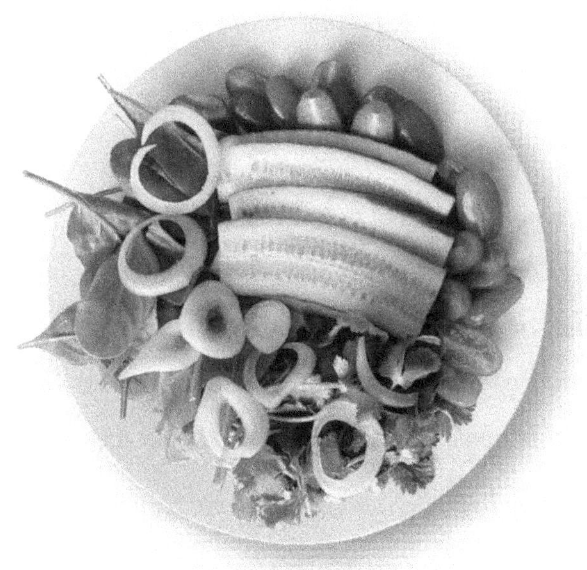

Simple Delicious and Healthy Recipes for Every Patient with Atrial Fibrillation to Promote Heart Health and Enhance Longevity Naturally (Cardiology Dietitian Guide)

Zeerah Amelia

TABLE OF CONTENTS

INTRODUCTION

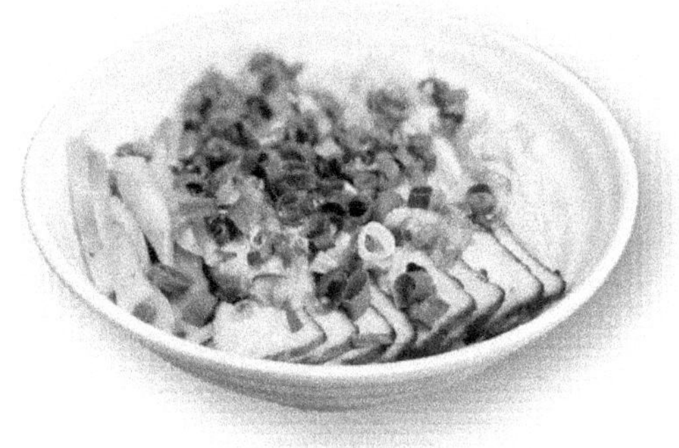

Atrial fibrillation (AFib) is a common irregular heart rhythm, known as an arrhythmia, that can lead to serious complications like stroke and heart failure. During AFib, the heart's upper chambers, called the atria, beat irregularly and out of sync with the lower chambers, known as the ventricles.

While some people may not experience symptoms, others may feel a fast, pounding heartbeat, shortness of breath, or dizziness. AFib can be occasional or ongoing and requires proper treatment, including a heart-healthy diet, to prevent complications.

AFib affects millions of people worldwide, including up to 6 million adults in the United States alone. It's the most common type of heart arrhythmia and increases the risk of death and disability.

Additionally, individuals with AFib may also experience a related condition called atrial flutter, which shares similar treatment approaches. AFib disrupts the heart's rhythm and can have serious health implications, emphasizing the importance of proper management and care.

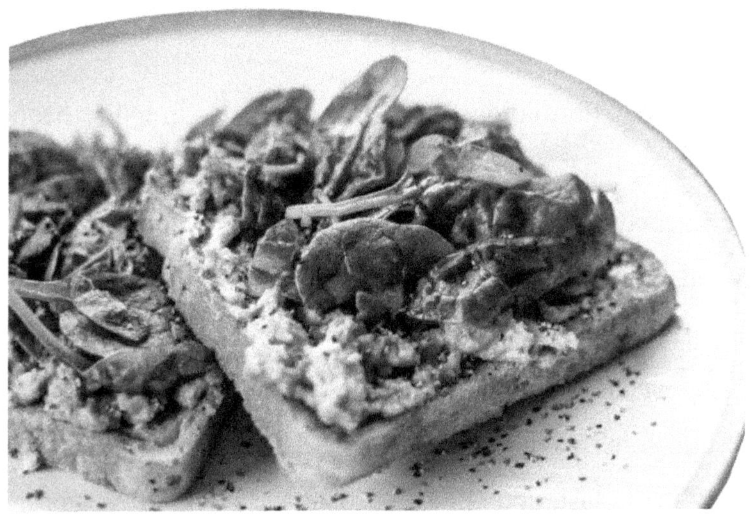

GETTING STARTED

"If you have been diagnosed with Atrial Fibrillation (AFib), you may be seeking natural ways to manage or potentially reverse it. Fortunately, *"The Complete AFib Diet Cookbook for Seniors"* offers dietary tips and recipes featuring heart-healthy ingredients carefully selected to manage and reverse Atrial Fibrillation and maintain overall cardiovascular health."

Each recipe in this cookbook includes:

- ✓ Accurate preparation times and servings
- ✓ Cook time estimates
- ✓ Budget-friendly ingredients
- ✓ Step-by-step cooking directions
- ✓ Nutritional values per serving
- ✓ Grocery shopping lists
- ✓ Ingredient substitution options

FOODS TO EAT:

- **Fruits and Vegetables:** Rich in vitamins, minerals, and antioxidants, they support heart health and overall well-being.

- **Whole Grains:** Provide fiber, vitamins, and minerals essential for heart health. Examples include quinoa, oats, brown rice, and whole wheat products.

- **Lean Proteins:** Opt for lean sources such as poultry, fish (especially fatty fish like salmon), tofu, beans, and legumes.

- **Healthy Fats:** Incorporate sources like avocados, nuts, seeds, and olive oil, which are rich in monounsaturated and polyunsaturated fats.

- **Omega-3 Fatty Acids:** Found in fatty fish, flaxseeds, chia seeds, and walnuts, they have anti-inflammatory properties beneficial for heart health.

- **Potassium-Rich Foods:** Bananas, oranges, spinach, sweet potatoes, and tomatoes help regulate blood pressure and heart rhythm.

- **Magnesium-Rich Foods:** Almonds, spinach, pumpkin seeds, and dark chocolate support heart function and rhythm regulation.

FOODS TO LIMIT OR AVOID:

- **Sodium:** Reduce intake of processed and packaged foods, as well as salty snacks, to help manage blood pressure and fluid retention.

- **Caffeine:** Limit consumption of coffee, tea, and caffeinated beverages, as they may trigger AFib episodes in some individuals.

- **Alcohol:** Limit or avoid alcohol, as it can increase the risk of AFib episodes and exacerbate symptoms.

- **Processed and Fried Foods:** Minimize consumption of processed meats, fried foods, and foods high in trans fats, which contribute to inflammation and heart disease risk.

- **Added Sugars:** Reduce intake of sugary snacks, desserts, and sweetened beverages, as they can lead to weight gain and heart health issues.

- **High-Fat Foods:** Limit saturated and trans fats found in fatty meats, full-fat dairy products, butter, and fried foods, as they can increase cholesterol levels and heart disease risk.

By focusing on a balanced diet rich in whole foods while limiting processed and unhealthy options, individuals can effectively manage and potentially reverse atrial fibrillation while promoting overall heart health. It's essential to consult with healthcare professionals for personalized dietary recommendations based on individual health needs and goals.

These recipes were delicious, heart-healthy, easy to prepare, and made with ingredients that are easily accessible to seniors, helping to promote longevity without straining finances."

BREAKFAST

1. Oatmeal with Berries

Prep time: 5 minutes

Cook time: 5 minutes

Ingredients:

- 1/2 cup rolled oats
- 1 cup water or low-fat milk
- 1/2 cup mixed berries (such as strawberries, blueberries, or raspberries)

Instructions:

- In a small saucepan, bring water or milk to a boil.
- Stir in the rolled oats and reduce heat to a simmer.

- Cook for about 5 minutes or until oats are tender and have absorbed most of the liquid.
- Serve hot, topped with mixed berries.

Nutritional information:

- Calories: 250
- Protein: 7g
- Carbohydrates: 45g
- Fat: 4g

Ingredient substitutions:

- Substitute rolled oats with instant oats for quicker cooking.
- Use frozen berries if fresh ones are not available.

2. Yogurt Parfait with Nuts

Prep time: 5 minutes

Ingredients:

- 1/2 cup low-fat yogurt
- 1/4 cup granola
- 1/4 cup mixed nuts (such as almonds, walnuts, or pecans)

Instructions:

- In a serving glass or bowl, layer the low-fat yogurt, granola, and mixed nuts.
- Repeat the layers until the ingredients are used up.
- Serve immediately.

Nutritional information:

- Calories: 300
- Protein: 10g
- Carbohydrates: 25g
- Fat: 18g

Ingredient substitutions:

- Substitute low-fat yogurt with Greek yogurt for added protein.
- Use your favorite type of nuts or seeds.

3. Whole Wheat Toast with Avocado

Prep time: 5 minutes

Ingredients:

- 2 slices whole wheat bread
- 1 ripe avocado

Instructions:

- Toast the whole wheat bread slices until golden brown.

- Mash the ripe avocado and spread it evenly on the toasted bread slices.
- Serve immediately.

Nutritional information:

- Calories: 280
- Protein: 7g
- Carbohydrates: 30g
- Fat: 16g

Ingredient substitutions:

- Add a sprinkle of sea salt or red pepper flakes for extra flavor.
- Substitute whole wheat bread with multigrain bread for added variety.

4. Fruit Smoothie

Prep time: 5 minutes

Ingredients:

- 1 ripe banana
- 1/2 cup frozen mixed berries
- 1/2 cup low-fat milk or almond milk

Instructions:

- In a blender, combine the ripe banana, frozen mixed berries, and low-fat milk.

- Blend until smooth and creamy.

- Pour into a glass and serve immediately.

Nutritional information:

- Calories: 200

- Protein: 5g

- Carbohydrates: 40g

- Fat: 2g

Ingredient substitutions:

- Use fresh fruits instead of frozen ones.

- Substitute milk with yogurt for a thicker consistency.

5. Vegetable Omelette

Prep time: 5 minutes

Cook time: 7 minutes

Ingredients:

- 2 eggs

- 1/4 cup diced vegetables (such as bell peppers, spinach, tomatoes)

Instructions:

- In a bowl, whisk the eggs until well beaten.
- Heat a non-stick skillet over medium heat and coat with cooking spray.
- Pour the beaten eggs into the skillet and swirl to coat the bottom evenly.
- Sprinkle the diced vegetables evenly over the eggs.
- Cook until the edges are set and the bottom is golden brown, then flip and cook the other side until cooked through.
- Slide the omelette onto a plate and serve hot.

Nutritional information:

- Calories: 220
- Protein: 14g
- Carbohydrates: 5g
- Fat: 15g

Ingredient substitutions:

- Add lean protein like turkey or chicken breast for added nutrition.
- Use any preferred vegetables or herbs for variety.

LUNCH

1. Quinoa Salad with Chickpeas

Prep time: 10 minutes

Cook time: 15 minutes (for quinoa)

Ingredients:

- 1/2 cup cooked quinoa
- 1/2 cup canned chickpeas, rinsed and drained
- 1/4 cup diced cucumber
- 1/4 cup cherry tomatoes, halved
- 2 tablespoons chopped fresh parsley
- 1 tablespoon olive oil
- 1 tablespoon lemon juice
- Salt and pepper to taste

Instructions:

- In a bowl, combine cooked quinoa, chickpeas, diced cucumber, cherry tomatoes, and chopped parsley.
- Drizzle olive oil and lemon juice over the salad.
- Season with salt and pepper, then toss gently to combine.
- Serve chilled or at room temperature.

Nutritional information:

- Calories: 320

- Protein: 10g

- Carbohydrates: 45g

- Fat: 12g

Ingredient substitutions:

- Substitute quinoa with brown rice or barley for a different grain base.

- Add other vegetables like bell peppers or red onions for more variety.

2. Tuna Salad Wrap

Prep time: 10 minutes

Ingredients:

- 1 small can (5 oz) tuna, drained

- 2 tablespoons Greek yogurt

- 1/4 cup diced celery

- 1/4 cup shredded carrots

- 2 whole wheat tortillas

Instructions:

- In a bowl, mix together tuna, Greek yogurt, diced celery, and shredded carrots until well combined.

- Divide the tuna salad mixture evenly between the two whole wheat tortillas.
- Roll up the tortillas, enclosing the filling tightly.
- Cut each wrap in half and serve.

Nutritional information:

- Calories: 300
- Protein: 25g
- Carbohydrates: 30g
- Fat: 10g

Ingredient substitutions:

- Substitute Greek yogurt with mayonnaise or avocado for a different flavor.
- Use lettuce leaves or spinach wraps for a lower-carb option.

3. Vegetable Stir-Fry with Brown Rice

Prep time: 10 minutes

Cook time: 15 minutes

Ingredients:

- 1 cup mixed vegetables (such as bell peppers, broccoli, carrots, snap peas)
- 1 tablespoon olive oil

- 2 cloves garlic, minced

- 2 cups cooked brown rice

- 2 tablespoons low-sodium soy sauce

Instructions:

- Heat olive oil in a large skillet over medium-high heat.

- Add minced garlic and stir-fry for 30 seconds.

- Add mixed vegetables and cook until tender-crisp, about 5-7 minutes.

- Add cooked brown rice and soy sauce to the skillet, stirring to combine.

- Cook for an additional 2-3 minutes until heated through.

- Serve hot.

Nutritional information:

- Calories: 350

- Protein: 8g

- Carbohydrates: 55g

- Fat: 10g

Ingredient substitutions:

- Use quinoa or quinoa/brown rice blend instead of plain brown rice.

- Add tofu or lean chicken breast for extra protein.

4. Turkey and Avocado Sandwich

Prep time: 10 minutes

Ingredients:

- 2 slices whole grain bread

- 3 slices lean turkey breast

- 1/4 avocado, sliced

- Handful of spinach leaves

Instructions:

- Toast the whole grain bread slices, if desired.

- Layer the slices of lean turkey breast, sliced avocado, and spinach leaves between the bread slices.

- Cut the sandwich in half and serve.

Nutritional information:

- Calories: 280

- Protein: 20g

- Carbohydrates: 30g

- Fat: 10g

Ingredient substitutions:

- Use multigrain bread or whole wheat wraps for variety.

- Add sliced tomatoes or cucumbers for extra crunch.

5. Mediterranean Chickpea Salad

Prep time: 10 minutes

Ingredients:

- 1 can (15 oz) chickpeas, rinsed and drained
- 1/4 cup diced cucumber
- 1/4 cup diced tomatoes
- 2 tablespoons chopped fresh parsley
- 2 tablespoons crumbled feta cheese
- 1 tablespoon olive oil
- 1 tablespoon lemon juice
- Salt and pepper to taste

Instructions:

- In a large bowl, combine chickpeas, diced cucumber, diced tomatoes, chopped parsley, and crumbled feta cheese.
- Drizzle olive oil and lemon juice over the salad.
- Season with salt and pepper, then toss gently to combine.
- Serve chilled or at room temperature.

Nutritional information:

- Calories: 320
- Protein: 12g

- Carbohydrates: 45g

- Fat: 12g

Ingredient substitutions:

- Add chopped olives or red onions for extra flavor.

- Substitute feta cheese with goat cheese or omit for a vegan option.

DINNER

1. Grilled Salmon with Asparagus

Prep time: 10 minutes

Cook time: 15 minutes

Ingredients:

- 2 salmon fillets (6 oz each)

- 1 bunch asparagus, trimmed

- 2 tablespoons olive oil

- Salt and pepper to taste

Instructions:

- Preheat grill to medium-high heat.

- Drizzle olive oil over salmon fillets and asparagus, then season with salt and pepper.

- Place salmon fillets and asparagus on the grill.
- Grill salmon for about 5-7 minutes on each side, or until fish flakes easily with a fork.
- Grill asparagus for about 5-8 minutes, or until tender.
- Serve hot.

Nutritional information:

- Calories: 350
- Protein: 30g
- Carbohydrates: 6g
- Fat: 22g

Ingredient substitutions:

- Substitute salmon with another fish like trout or tilapia.
- Replace asparagus with green beans or zucchini.

2. Quinoa Stuffed Bell Peppers

Prep time: 15 minutes

Cook time: 30 minutes

Ingredients:

- 4 bell peppers, tops removed and seeded
- 1 cup cooked quinoa
- 1 can (15 oz) black beans, rinsed and drained

- 1 cup corn kernels

- 1 cup diced tomatoes

- 1 teaspoon cumin

- 1/2 teaspoon chili powder

- Salt and pepper to taste

Instructions:

- Preheat oven to 375°F (190°C).

- In a large bowl, combine cooked quinoa, black beans, corn kernels, diced tomatoes, cumin, chili powder, salt, and pepper.

- Stuff each bell pepper with the quinoa mixture.

- Place stuffed bell peppers in a baking dish and cover with foil.

- Bake for 25-30 minutes, or until peppers are tender.

- Serve hot.

Nutritional information:

- Calories: 280

- Protein: 10g

- Carbohydrates: 50g

- Fat: 4g

Ingredient substitutions:

- Substitute quinoa with brown rice or couscous.

- Add diced onions or mushrooms for extra flavor.

3. Chicken and Vegetable Stir-Fry

Prep time: 15 minutes

Cook time: 15 minutes

Ingredients:

- 2 boneless, skinless chicken breasts, thinly sliced

- 2 cups mixed vegetables (such as bell peppers, broccoli, carrots, snap peas)

- 2 tablespoons soy sauce

- 1 tablespoon olive oil

- 2 cloves garlic, minced

- 1 teaspoon ginger, minced

- Cooked brown rice or quinoa for serving

Instructions:

- Heat olive oil in a large skillet or wok over medium-high heat.

- Add minced garlic and ginger, and stir-fry for 30 seconds.

- Add sliced chicken breasts to the skillet and cook until browned and cooked through, about 5-7 minutes.

- Add mixed vegetables to the skillet and stir-fry until tender-crisp, about 5 minutes.
- Pour soy sauce over the chicken and vegetables, stirring to combine.
- Serve hot over cooked brown rice or quinoa.

Nutritional information:

- Calories: 320
- Protein: 30g
- Carbohydrates: 20g
- Fat: 12g

Ingredient substitutions:

- Use shrimp or tofu instead of chicken.
- Add your favorite stir-fry sauce for extra flavor.

4. Vegetarian Chili

Prep time: 15 minutes

Cook time: 30 minutes

Ingredients:

- 1 can (15 oz) black beans, rinsed and drained
- 1 can (15 oz) kidney beans, rinsed and drained
- 1 can (15 oz) diced tomatoes

- 1 cup corn kernels
- 1 bell pepper, diced
- 1 onion, diced
- 2 cloves garlic, minced
- 1 tablespoon chili powder
- 1 teaspoon cumin
- Salt and pepper to taste

Instructions:

- In a large pot, heat olive oil over medium heat.
- Add diced onion and bell pepper, and cook until softened, about 5 minutes.
- Add minced garlic, chili powder, cumin, salt, and pepper, and cook for 1 minute.
- Add black beans, kidney beans, diced tomatoes, and corn kernels to the pot.
- Bring the chili to a simmer and let it cook for 20-25 minutes, stirring occasionally.
- Serve hot, optionally topped with shredded cheese or a dollop of Greek yogurt.

Nutritional information:

- Calories: 300
- Protein: 15g

- Carbohydrates: 55g

- Fat: 2g

Ingredient substitutions:

- Add diced carrots or sweet potatoes for extra sweetness and nutrients.

- Use vegetable broth instead of water for a richer flavor.

5. Mushroom and Spinach Pasta

Prep time: 15 minutes

Cook time: 20 minutes

Ingredients:

- 8 oz whole wheat pasta

- 2 cups sliced mushrooms

- 2 cups baby spinach leaves

- 2 cloves garlic, minced

- 1 tablespoon olive oil

- 1/4 cup grated Parmesan cheese

- Salt and pepper to taste

Instructions:

- Cook pasta according to package instructions until al dente. Drain and set aside.

- In a large skillet, heat olive oil over medium heat.

- Add minced garlic and sliced mushrooms to the skillet, and cook until mushrooms are tender, about 5 minutes.

- Add baby spinach leaves to the skillet and cook until wilted, about 2 minutes.

- Add cooked pasta to the skillet and toss to combine.

- Season with salt and pepper, and sprinkle grated Parmesan cheese over the pasta.

- Serve hot.

Nutritional information:

- Calories: 350

- Protein: 12g

- Carbohydrates: 50g

- Fat: 10g

Ingredient substitutions:

- Use any type of pasta you prefer, such as penne or spaghetti.

- Add diced tomatoes or sun-dried tomatoes for extra flavor and color.

1. Banana Walnut Oatmeal

Prep time: 5 minutes

Cook time: 10 minutes

Servings: 1

Ingredients:

- 1 ripe banana, mashed
- 1/2 cup rolled oats
- 1 cup unsweetened almond milk
- 1 tablespoon chopped walnuts

Instructions:

- In a small saucepan, bring almond milk to a gentle boil.
- Stir in rolled oats and reduce heat to low. Cook for 5-7 minutes, stirring occasionally until oats are tender and mixture thickens.
- Remove from heat and stir in mashed banana.
- Serve hot, topped with chopped walnuts.

Nutritional value (per serving):

- Calories: 320
- Protein: 9g
- Fat: 10g
- Carbohydrates: 54g
- Fiber: 7g

Ingredient substitutions:

- Substitute almond milk with any other plant-based milk.
- Use chopped almonds or pecans instead of walnuts.

2. Greek Yogurt with Berries

Prep time: 3 minutes

Servings: 1

Ingredients:

- 1/2 cup plain Greek yogurt
- 1/2 cup mixed berries (such as strawberries, blueberries, raspberries)

Instructions:

- In a serving bowl, spoon Greek yogurt.
- Top with mixed berries.
- Serve chilled.

Nutritional value (per serving):

- Calories: 120
- Protein: 17g
- Fat: 0.5g
- Carbohydrates: 15g
- Fiber: 3g

Ingredient substitutions:

- Use dairy-free yogurt for a vegan option.

- Add a drizzle of honey or maple syrup for sweetness if desired.

3. Avocado Toast with Tomato

Prep time: 5 minutes

Servings: 1

Ingredients:

- 1 slice whole grain bread, toasted
- 1/2 ripe avocado, mashed
- 1 small tomato, sliced
- Pinch of black pepper

Instructions:

- Spread mashed avocado evenly on the toasted bread slice.
- Top with sliced tomato.
- Sprinkle black pepper on top.
- Serve immediately.

Nutritional value (per serving):

- Calories: 200
- Protein: 5g
- Fat: 10g
- Carbohydrates: 23g
- Fiber: 7g

Ingredient substitutions:

- Use multigrain or seeded bread for added fiber and nutrients.

- Add a dash of lemon juice or balsamic vinegar for extra flavor.

4. Tuna Salad Lettuce Wraps

Prep time: 10 minutes

Servings: 2

Ingredients:

- 1 can (5 oz) tuna in water, drained
- 2 tablespoons plain Greek yogurt
- 1 tablespoon lemon juice
- 1/4 cup diced cucumber
- 1/4 cup diced bell pepper
- 4 large lettuce leaves (such as romaine or butter lettuce)

Instructions:

- In a bowl, combine tuna, Greek yogurt, lemon juice, cucumber, and bell pepper. Mix well.
- Spoon tuna salad mixture onto lettuce leaves.
- Wrap lettuce around the filling.
- Serve immediately.

Nutritional value (per serving, 2 wraps):

- Calories: 120
- Protein: 14g
- Fat: 3g
- Carbohydrates: 7g
- Fiber: 2g

Ingredient substitutions:

- Use canned salmon instead of tuna for variation.
- Add diced celery or carrots for extra crunch and nutrients.

5. Fruit and Nut Trail Mix

Prep time: 2 minutes

Servings: 1

Ingredients:

- 1/4 cup mixed nuts (almonds, walnuts, cashews)
- 1/4 cup dried fruit (raisins, cranberries, apricots)
- **Instructions:**
- In a bowl, combine mixed nuts and dried fruit.
- Mix well.
- Portion into a snack-sized container for easy grab-and-go access.

Nutritional value (per serving):

- Calories: 200
- Protein: 5g
- Fat: 12g
- Carbohydrates: 20g
- Fiber: 4g

Ingredient substitutions:

- Use seeds like pumpkin or sunflower seeds as a nut alternative.

- Choose unsweetened dried fruit to limit added sugars.

DESSERTS

1. Baked Apple with Cinnamon

Prep time: 5 minutes

Cook time: 25 minutes

Servings: 2

Ingredients:

- 2 apples, cored and halved
- 1 teaspoon cinnamon
- 1 tablespoon chopped walnuts (optional)

Instructions:

- Preheat the oven to 375°F (190°C).
- Place the apple halves on a baking sheet lined with parchment paper.
- Sprinkle cinnamon evenly over the apple halves.
- Optionally, sprinkle chopped walnuts over the apples.
- Bake in the preheated oven for 20-25 minutes, or until the apples are tender.
- Remove from the oven and let cool slightly before serving.

Nutritional value (per serving):

- Calories: 90

- Protein: 1g
- Fat: 1g
- Carbohydrates: 25g
- Fiber: 5g

Ingredient substitutions:

- Use pears instead of apples for variety.
- Add a drizzle of honey or maple syrup for extra sweetness if desired.

2. Chia Seed Pudding

Prep time: 5 minutes (+ chilling time)

Servings: 2

Ingredients:

- 1/4 cup chia seeds
- 1 cup unsweetened almond milk
- 1 tablespoon maple syrup or honey (optional)
- 1/2 teaspoon vanilla extract

Instructions:

- In a bowl, whisk together chia seeds, almond milk, maple syrup or honey (if using), and vanilla extract.
- Let the mixture sit for 5 minutes, then whisk again to prevent clumping.
- Cover and refrigerate for at least 2 hours or overnight, until the mixture thickens into pudding-like consistency.

- Stir well before serving and add toppings if desired, such as fresh berries or sliced almonds.

Nutritional value (per serving):

- Calories: 130
- Protein: 4g
- Fat: 7g
- Carbohydrates: 15g
- Fiber: 9g

Ingredient substitutions:

- Use any other type of milk (such as coconut milk or cow's milk) instead of almond milk.
- Experiment with different flavorings like cocoa powder or almond extract.

3. Frozen Banana Bites

Prep time: 10 minutes (+ freezing time)

Servings: 2

Ingredients:

- 1 ripe banana, sliced into rounds
- 2 tablespoons almond butter
- 2 tablespoons unsweetened shredded coconut (optional)

Instructions:

- Spread almond butter on half of the banana slices.
- Top each almond butter-covered slice with another banana slice to form sandwiches.

- Roll the edges of each banana sandwich in shredded coconut if desired.
- Place the banana bites on a parchment-lined baking sheet and freeze for at least 2 hours until firm.
- Serve frozen as a refreshing dessert or snack.

Nutritional value (per serving):

- Calories: 180
- Protein: 3g
- Fat: 10g
- Carbohydrates: 20g
- Fiber: 4g

Ingredient substitutions:

- Use peanut butter or any other nut butter of your choice.
- Roll the edges of the banana bites in chopped nuts instead of shredded coconut for added crunch.

4. Dark Chocolate Covered Strawberries

Prep time: 15 minutes (+ chilling time)

Servings: 2

Ingredients:

- 6 large strawberries, washed and dried
- 2 ounces dark chocolate (70% cocoa or higher), chopped
- 1 teaspoon coconut oil

- Optional toppings: chopped nuts, shredded coconut

Instructions:

- Line a baking sheet with parchment paper.
- In a heatproof bowl, combine the chopped dark chocolate and coconut oil.
- Microwave in 30-second intervals, stirring in between, until the chocolate is melted and smooth.
- Holding each strawberry by the stem, dip it into the melted chocolate, coating it halfway.
- Place the dipped strawberries on the prepared baking sheet.
- Optional: sprinkle chopped nuts or shredded coconut over the chocolate-coated part of the strawberries.
- Refrigerate for at least 30 minutes, or until the chocolate is set.
- Serve chilled.

Nutritional value (per serving):

- Calories: 120
- Protein: 1g
- Fat: 8g
- Carbohydrates: 13g
- Fiber: 3g

Ingredient substitutions:

- Use milk or white chocolate if preferred, but opt for those with higher cocoa content for better heart health benefits.
- Swap coconut oil with vegetable oil if needed.

5. Baked Pears with Cinnamon and Honey

Prep time: 10 minutes

Cook time: 25 minutes

Servings: 2

Ingredients:

- 2 ripe pears, halved and cored
- 1 tablespoon honey
- 1/2 teaspoon cinnamon
- Optional toppings: chopped nuts, Greek yogurt

Instructions:

- Preheat the oven to 375°F (190°C).
- Place the pear halves, cut side up, on a baking dish.
- Drizzle honey over the pear halves and sprinkle with cinnamon.
- Bake in the preheated oven for 20-25 minutes, or until the pears are tender.
- Remove from the oven and let cool slightly before serving.
- Optionally, serve with a dollop of Greek yogurt and sprinkle with chopped nuts.

Nutritional value (per serving):

- Calories: 120
- Protein: 1g
- Fat: 0g
- Carbohydrates: 30g

- Fiber: 5g

Ingredient substitutions:

- Use maple syrup instead of honey for a vegan option.
- Top with granola instead of chopped nuts for added texture.

SMOOTHIES

1. Berry Green Smoothie

Prep time: 5 minutes

Servings: 2

Ingredients:

- 1 cup spinach leaves, packed
- 1/2 cup frozen mixed berries (strawberries, blueberries, raspberries)
- 1 ripe banana
- 1 cup unsweetened almond milk
- 1 tablespoon chia seeds (optional)

Instructions:

- In a blender, combine spinach, mixed berries, banana, almond milk, and chia seeds (if using).
- Blend until smooth and creamy.
- If the smoothie is too thick, add more almond milk until desired consistency is reached.
- Pour into glasses and serve immediately.

Nutritional value (per serving):

- Calories: 120
- Protein: 3g
- Fat: 4g
- Carbohydrates: 22g
- Fiber: 6g

Ingredient substitutions:

- Use kale or Swiss chard instead of spinach for variation.
- Substitute any other type of milk (such as coconut milk or cow's milk) for almond milk.

2. Tropical Mango Smoothie

Prep time: 5 minutes

Servings: 2

Ingredients:

- 1 ripe mango, peeled and diced
- 1/2 cup pineapple chunks (fresh or frozen)
- 1/2 cup plain Greek yogurt
- 1/2 cup unsweetened coconut water
- 1 tablespoon honey (optional)

Instructions:

- In a blender, combine diced mango, pineapple chunks, Greek yogurt, coconut water, and honey (if using).
- Blend until smooth and creamy.

- If the smoothie is too thick, add more coconut water until desired consistency is reached.
- Pour into glasses and serve immediately.

Nutritional value (per serving):

- Calories: 150
- Protein: 6g
- Fat: 1g
- Carbohydrates: 32g
- Fiber: 3g

Ingredient substitutions:

- Use frozen banana instead of Greek yogurt for a dairy-free option.
- Substitute orange juice for coconut water for a different flavor profile.

3. Banana Peanut Butter Smoothie

Prep time: 5 minutes

Servings: 2

Ingredients:

- 2 ripe bananas
- 2 tablespoons peanut butter (unsweetened)
- 1 cup unsweetened almond milk
- 1 tablespoon flaxseeds (optional)
- Ice cubes (optional)

Instructions:

- In a blender, combine ripe bananas, peanut butter, almond milk, and flaxseeds (if using).
- Add ice cubes if desired for a colder smoothie.
- Blend until smooth and creamy.
- Adjust the consistency by adding more almond milk if needed.
- Pour into glasses and serve immediately.

Nutritional value (per serving):

- Calories: 250
- Protein: 7g
- Fat: 13g
- Carbohydrates: 30g
- Fiber: 5g

Ingredient substitutions:

- Use any other nut or seed butter such as almond butter or sunflower seed butter.
- Substitute dairy milk or soy milk for almond milk if preferred.

4. Spinach Avocado Smoothie

Prep time: 5 minutes

Servings: 2

Ingredients:

- 2 cups fresh spinach leaves, packed
- 1 ripe avocado, peeled and pitted

- 1 cup unsweetened coconut water
- Juice of 1 lime
- 1 tablespoon honey or maple syrup (optional)

Instructions:

- In a blender, combine fresh spinach leaves, ripe avocado, coconut water, lime juice, and honey or maple syrup (if using).
- Blend until smooth and creamy.
- Adjust sweetness by adding more honey or maple syrup if desired.
- Pour into glasses and serve immediately.

Nutritional value (per serving):

- Calories: 180
- Protein: 3g
- Fat: 10g
- Carbohydrates: 22g
- Fiber: 9g

Ingredient substitutions:

- Substitute kale or Swiss chard for spinach for a different flavor profile.
- Use lemon juice instead of lime juice if preferred.

5. Blueberry Almond Smoothie

Prep time: 5 minutes

Servings: 2

Ingredients:

- 1 cup frozen blueberries
- 1/4 cup almonds
- 1 ripe banana
- 1 cup unsweetened almond milk
- 1 tablespoon honey or maple syrup (optional)

Instructions:

- In a blender, combine frozen blueberries, almonds, ripe banana, almond milk, and honey or maple syrup (if using).
- Blend until smooth and creamy.
- Adjust sweetness by adding more honey or maple syrup if desired.
- Pour into glasses and serve immediately.

Nutritional value (per serving):

- Calories: 220
- Protein: 5g
- Fat: 10g
- Carbohydrates: 30g
- Fiber: 6g

Ingredient substitutions:

- Use any other type of berry such as strawberries or raspberries.
- Substitute almond milk with any other milk alternative such as soy milk or oat milk.

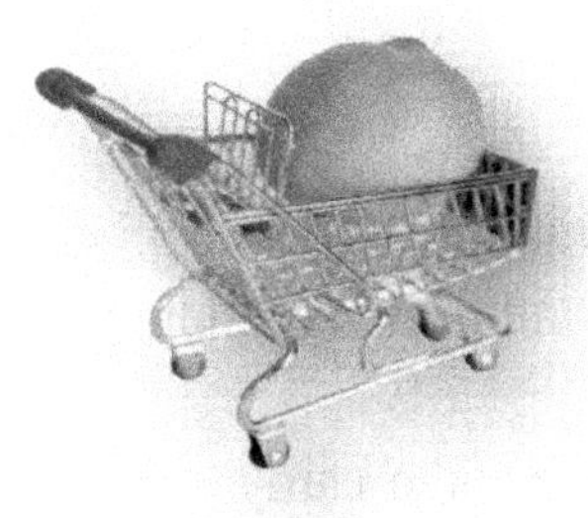

BREAKFAST:

1. Oatmeal with Berries:

- Rolled oats
- Mixed berries (strawberries, blueberries, raspberries)
- Low-fat milk or water

2. Yogurt Parfait with Nuts:

- Low-fat yogurt
- Granola
- Mixed nuts (almonds, walnuts, pecans)

3. Whole Wheat Toast with Avocado:

- Whole wheat bread
- Ripe avocado

4. Fruit Smoothie:

- Banana

- Mixed berries (strawberries, blueberries, raspberries)

- Low-fat milk or almond milk

5. Vegetable Omelette:

- Eggs

- Diced vegetables (bell peppers, spinach, tomatoes)

LUNCH:

1. Quinoa Salad with Chickpeas:

- Quinoa

- Canned chickpeas

- Cucumber

- Cherry tomatoes

- Parsley

2. Tuna Salad Wrap:

- Tuna

- Greek yogurt

- Celery

- Carrots

- Whole wheat tortillas

3. Vegetable Stir-Fry with Brown Rice:

- Mixed vegetables (bell peppers, broccoli, carrots, snap peas)
- Brown rice
- Garlic
- Soy sauce

4. Turkey and Avocado Sandwich:

- Whole grain bread
- Turkey breast slices
- Avocado
- Spinach leaves

5. Mediterranean Chickpea Salad:

- Chickpeas
- Cucumber
- Tomatoes
- Parsley
- Feta cheese

DINNER:

1. Grilled Salmon with Asparagus:

- Salmon fillets
- Asparagus
- Olive oil

2. Quinoa Stuffed Bell Peppers:

- Bell peppers
- Quinoa
- Black beans
- Corn kernels
- Diced tomatoes

3. Chicken and Vegetable Stir-Fry:

- Chicken breasts
- Mixed vegetables (bell peppers, broccoli, carrots, snap peas)
- Brown rice or quinoa

4. Vegetarian Chili:

- Black beans
- Kidney beans
- Diced tomatoes

- Corn kernels

- Onion

- Garlic

- Chili powder

5. *Mushroom and Spinach Pasta:*

- Whole wheat pasta

- Mushrooms

- Spinach

- Garlic

- Parmesan cheese

SNACKS:

1. *Banana Walnut Oatmeal:*

- Ripe banana

- Rolled oats

- Unsweetened almond milk

- Chopped walnuts

2. *Greek Yogurt with Berries:*

- Plain Greek yogurt

- Mixed berries (strawberries, blueberries, raspberries)

3. Avocado Toast with Tomato:

- Whole grain bread

- Ripe avocado

- Tomato

- Black pepper

4. Tuna Salad Lettuce Wraps:

- Canned tuna in water
- Plain Greek yogurt
- Lemon
- Cucumber
- Bell pepper
- Lettuce leaves (romaine or butter lettuce)

5. Fruit and Nut Trail Mix:

- Mixed nuts (almonds, walnuts, cashews)

- Dried fruit (raisins, cranberries, apricots)

DESSERTS:

1. Baked Apple with Cinnamon:

- Apples

- Cinnamon

- Chopped walnuts (optional)

2. *Chia Seed Pudding:*

- Chia seeds

- Unsweetened almond milk

- Maple syrup or honey

- Vanilla extract

3. *Frozen Banana Bites:*

- Ripe bananas

- Almond butter

- Unsweetened shredded coconut (optional)

4. *Dark Chocolate Covered Strawberries:*

- Large strawberries

- Dark chocolate (70% cocoa or higher)

- Coconut oil

- Optional toppings: chopped nuts, shredded coconut

5. *Baked Pears with Cinnamon and Honey:*

- Ripe pears

- Honey

- Cinnamon

- Optional toppings: chopped nuts, Greek yogurt

SMOOTHIES:

1. Berry Green Smoothie:

- Spinach leaves
- Frozen mixed berries
- Ripe banana
- Unsweetened almond milk
- Chia seeds (optional)

2. Tropical Mango Smoothie:

- Ripe mango
- Pineapple chunks
- Plain Greek yogurt
- Unsweetened coconut water
- Honey (optional)

3. Banana Peanut Butter Smoothie:

- Ripe bananas
- Peanut butter (unsweetened)
- Unsweetened almond milk
- Flaxseeds (optional)
- Ice cubes (optional)

4. Spinach Avocado Smoothie:

- Fresh spinach leaves

- Ripe avocado

- Unsweetened coconut water

- Lime

- Honey or maple syrup (optional)

5. Blueberry Almond Smoothie:

- Frozen blueberries
- Almonds
- Ripe banana
- Unsweetened almond milk
- Honey or maple syrup (optional)

Make sure to adjust quantities based on the number of servings you intend to prepare and any personal preferences. Happy shopping and cooking!

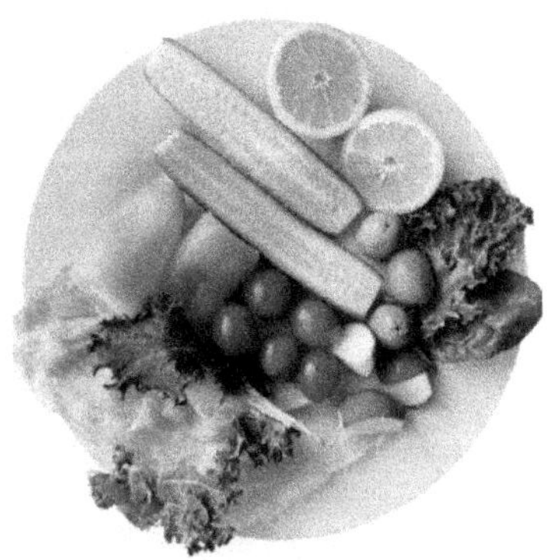

CONCLUSION

The Complete AFib Diet Cookbook for Seniors" serves as a valuable resource for individuals seeking to manage and improve their atrial fibrillation (AFib) through dietary strategies. This comprehensive cookbook provides seniors with delicious and nutritious recipes tailored to support heart health and manage AFib symptoms.

By emphasizing whole foods rich in fruits, vegetables, lean proteins, and healthy fats, this cookbook offers a roadmap for adopting a heart-healthy lifestyle. Through careful consideration of ingredients and cooking methods, seniors can cultivate habits that promote optimal cardiovascular function and overall well-being.

Moreover, the cookbook recognizes the importance of individualized dietary approaches and encourages readers to consult with healthcare professionals for personalized guidance. By incorporating the principles outlined in this cookbook into their daily routines, seniors can take proactive steps towards managing AFib and enhancing their quality of life. With its accessible recipes and evidence-based recommendations, "The Complete AFib Diet Cookbook for Seniors" empowers individuals to embrace delicious, nourishing meals that support heart health and vitality.

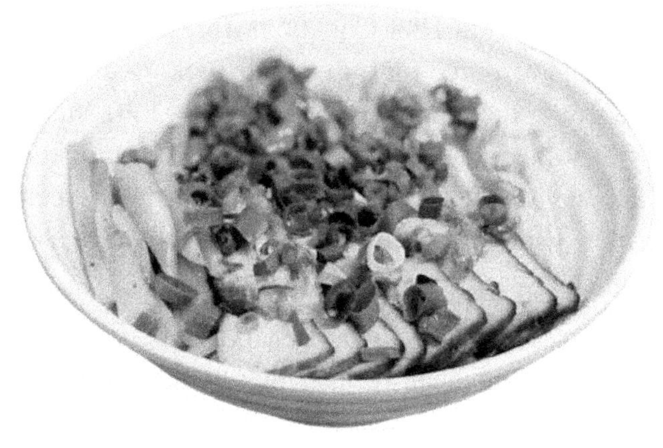

HAPPY

COOKING!

www.ingramcontent.com/pod-product-compliance
Lightning Source LLC
Chambersburg PA
CBHW061935270726
48660CB00007BA/2728